From Farm to Lab: The Role of Biotechnology in Agriculture and Food Production

Graham Max

Copyright © [2023]

Title: From Farm to Lab: The Role of Biotechnology in Agriculture and Food Production
Author's: Graham Max

All rights reserved. No part of this publication may be reproduced, stored in a retrieval system, or transmitted in any form or by any means, electronic, mechanical, photocopying, recording, or otherwise, without the prior written permission of the publisher or author, except in the case of brief quotations embodied in critical reviews and certain other non-commercial uses permitted by copyright law.

This book was printed and published by [Publisher's: **Graham Max**] in [2023]

ISBN:

TABLE OF CONTENT

Chapter 1: Introduction to Biotechnology in Agriculture and Food Production   07

The Evolution of Agriculture: From Traditional Farming to Modern Biotechnology

The Importance of Biotechnology in Food Production

The Purpose of this Book: Exploring the Role of Biotechnology in Agriculture

Chapter 2: Understanding Biotechnology in Agriculture   14

Defining Biotechnology and its Applications in Agriculture

Genetic Engineering: Manipulating Plant and Animal Genomes

Crop Improvement through Biotechnology

Livestock Biotechnology: Enhancing Animal Health and Productivity

## Chapter 3: Biotechnology and Crop Production	22

Overview of Biotech Crops: GM Crops and their Benefits

Herbicide Tolerance: Reducing Weed Pressure in Fields

Pest Resistance: Enhancing Crop Protection

Drought and Salinity Tolerance: Improving Crop Resilience

## Chapter 4: Biotechnology and Livestock Production	30

Animal Biotechnology: An Overview

Biotechnological Approaches to Enhancing Animal Health

Improving Animal Productivity through Biotechnology

Biotechnology and Animal Welfare

## Chapter 5: Biotechnology and Food Processing	38

Food Processing and Biotechnology: An Introduction

Microbial Biotechnology: Fermentation and Food Preservation

Genetic Modification in Food Processing: Enhancing Nutritional Value

Chapter 6: Biotechnology and Food Safety　　　　　　　　　　　45

Ensuring Food Safety: An Introduction to Biotechnology

Biotechnology and Foodborne Pathogens: Detection and Control

Controversies and Concerns: GMO Labeling and Consumer Awareness

Chapter 7: Biotechnology and Sustainable Agriculture　　　　　　　　　　　51

Sustainable Agriculture: An Overview

Biotechnology and Environmental Sustainability

Biotechnology and Resource Conservation

Biotechnology and Organic Farming

Chapter 8: Future Trends and Challenges in Biotechnology　　　　　　　　　　　60

Emerging Technologies in Biotechnology

Ethical Considerations in Biotechnology

Regulatory Frameworks: Balancing Innovation and Safety

Overcoming Challenges: Bridging the Gap between Science and Society

Chapter 9: Conclusion 68

Recapitulation of Key Points

The Future of Biotechnology in Agriculture and Food Production

Final Thoughts: Harnessing the Potential of Biotechnology for a Sustainable Future

Chapter 1: Introduction to Biotechnology in Agriculture and Food Production

The Evolution of Agriculture: From Traditional Farming to Modern Biotechnology

Introduction:
The history of agriculture is a testament to human innovation and adaptability. From the humble beginnings of traditional farming practices to the revolutionary advancements in modern biotechnology, the agricultural industry has undergone a remarkable transformation. In this subchapter, we will explore the fascinating journey of agriculture, tracing its roots back to ancient civilizations and delving into the groundbreaking developments that have shaped the field of biotechnology today.

Traditional Farming:
Traditional farming methods have been practiced for thousands of years, rooted in the knowledge and expertise of early farmers. These methods relied heavily on human labor, utilizing simple tools and techniques to cultivate crops and raise livestock. From hand planting and animal-powered plowing to crop rotation and selective breeding, traditional farming was a labor-intensive process that played a crucial role in sustaining human populations.

The Green Revolution:
The mid-20th century marked a turning point in agricultural history with the advent of the Green Revolution. This period saw the introduction of high-yielding crop varieties, synthetic fertilizers, and the widespread use of pesticides. These innovations significantly

increased crop productivity, allowing farmers to meet the growing demand for food. However, the Green Revolution also raised concerns about environmental sustainability and the long-term effects of chemical inputs on human health.

The Rise of Biotechnology:
In recent decades, biotechnology has emerged as a game-changer in the agricultural industry. By harnessing the power of genetic engineering, scientists have been able to develop crops with enhanced traits, such as disease resistance, improved nutritional content, and increased yield. Biotechnology has also enabled the development of genetically modified organisms (GMOs), which have sparked debates regarding their safety, ethics, and potential impact on biodiversity.

Benefits and Impact:
The integration of biotechnology in agriculture has brought forth numerous benefits. Improved crop varieties have increased productivity, reducing the reliance on chemical inputs and minimizing the environmental impact of farming practices. Biotechnology has also played a crucial role in addressing global challenges such as food security, climate change, and sustainable agriculture. However, it is essential to carefully assess the potential risks and ethical considerations associated with the use of biotechnology in agriculture.

Conclusion:
The evolution of agriculture from traditional farming to modern biotechnology has been a remarkable journey. The advancements in biotechnology have revolutionized crop production, allowing for increased yields, improved nutrition, and enhanced sustainability. However, it is important to strike a balance between the benefits and

potential risks associated with biotechnology. As we continue to explore the role of biotechnology in agriculture, it is crucial to engage in informed discussions and make responsible choices that ensure a sustainable future for our food production systems.

The Importance of Biotechnology in Food Production

In today's world, where the global population is rapidly increasing, ensuring food security has become a paramount concern. Biotechnology, a field that combines biology and technology, has emerged as a powerful tool in addressing this challenge. With its ability to enhance crop yield, improve nutritional content, and reduce environmental impact, biotechnology plays a crucial role in food production.

One of the primary contributions of biotechnology to food production is the development of genetically modified organisms (GMOs). By altering an organism's genetic makeup, scientists can create crops that are resistant to pests, diseases, and harsh environmental conditions. This not only increases yield but also reduces the need for harmful pesticides and herbicides, making agriculture more sustainable. GMOs have already made a significant impact by improving the productivity of staple crops like corn, soybean, and cotton.

Biotechnology also enables the development of crops with enhanced nutritional profiles. For example, through genetic engineering, scientists have successfully increased the vitamin A content in rice, addressing a prevalent deficiency known as "hidden hunger." Similarly, biotech crops can be fortified with essential minerals, vitamins, and proteins, ensuring a more balanced and nutritious diet for populations that rely heavily on these crops.

Furthermore, biotechnology plays a vital role in reducing post-harvest losses. By enhancing the shelf life of fruits and vegetables, biotech techniques such as genetic modification and preservation technologies help prevent spoilage and minimize waste. This is particularly crucial in regions where transportation and storage infrastructure are inadequate.

Biotechnology also contributes to sustainable agriculture practices. Through the use of biofertilizers and biopesticides, farmers can reduce their dependence on synthetic chemicals, minimizing environmental pollution. Additionally, biotechnology aids in the development of drought-tolerant and salt-tolerant crops, allowing farmers to cultivate in arid and saline regions that were previously unsuitable for agriculture.

In conclusion, biotechnology is revolutionizing food production by addressing the challenges of increasing global food demand, nutritional deficiencies, and environmental sustainability. By harnessing the power of genetic engineering and other innovative techniques, biotechnology has the potential to transform agriculture and ensure food security for present and future generations. Embracing biotechnology in food production is not only crucial for meeting the needs of a growing population but also for building a sustainable and healthy future for all.

The Purpose of this Book: Exploring the Role of Biotechnology in Agriculture

Welcome to "From Farm to Lab: The Role of Biotechnology in Agriculture and Food Production." This book aims to provide a comprehensive exploration of the fascinating field of biotechnology and its profound impact on agriculture. Whether you are a curious reader seeking to understand the intricacies of biotechnology or a professional in the fields of biomedical science and biotechnology, this book is designed to cater to your interests and knowledge.

In recent years, the world has witnessed an exponential growth in the application of biotechnology in agriculture. This emerging field has revolutionized food production, ensuring food security, and tackling various agricultural challenges. Through the integration of advanced genetic techniques, biotechnology has enhanced crop yields, increased resistance to pests and diseases, and improved nutritional content. It has also facilitated the development of genetically modified organisms (GMOs), which have sparked debates and discussions on their benefits and potential risks.

The main purpose of this book is to delve into the multifaceted role of biotechnology in agriculture. We will explore the scientific principles behind biotechnology and its practical applications in improving crop productivity, enhancing crop quality, and promoting sustainable farming practices. Furthermore, we will examine the ethical, social, and environmental implications associated with the adoption of biotechnology in agriculture.

Whether you are a student, researcher, or simply an individual interested in the future of agriculture, this book will provide you with a comprehensive understanding of the latest advancements in biotechnology and their implications for food production. With contributions from leading experts in the field, each chapter will present a balanced perspective on the potential benefits and challenges of biotechnology in agriculture.

Through engaging narratives, case studies, and up-to-date research findings, "From Farm to Lab: The Role of Biotechnology in Agriculture and Food Production" aims to inspire critical thinking and informed discussions around the role of biotechnology in shaping the future of agriculture. We invite you to embark on this enlightening journey, where science meets innovation, and explore the exciting possibilities that biotechnology holds for a sustainable and secure food system.

Join us as we unlock the mysteries of biotechnology and discover how it is transforming the way we produce and consume food.

Chapter 2: Understanding Biotechnology in Agriculture

Defining Biotechnology and its Applications in Agriculture

Biotechnology, an interdisciplinary field that combines biology and technology, has revolutionized various industries including agriculture. In this subchapter, we will delve into the concept of biotechnology and explore its wide-ranging applications in the agricultural sector.

Biotechnology can be defined as the use of living organisms or their products to modify or improve upon processes, products, or systems. In the context of agriculture, biotechnology encompasses the application of genetic engineering, molecular biology, and other techniques to enhance crop productivity, improve plant characteristics, and develop sustainable farming practices.

One of the major applications of biotechnology in agriculture is the development of genetically modified organisms (GMOs). GMOs are organisms whose genetic material has been altered in a way that does not occur naturally through mating or natural recombination. These genetically modified crops possess desirable traits such as resistance to pests, diseases, or herbicides, enabling farmers to achieve higher yields and reduce the use of chemical inputs. GMOs have found widespread adoption around the globe, contributing to increased food production and enhanced food security.

Additionally, biotechnology plays a vital role in improving crop quality and nutritional value. Scientists can use genetic engineering to enhance the nutritional content of crops, making them more resistant to nutrient deficiencies. For example, by introducing specific genes, scientists have developed biofortified crops that are enriched with essential vitamins and minerals, addressing malnutrition in vulnerable populations.

Biotechnology also aids in the development of sustainable farming practices. Through bioremediation, microorganisms are utilized to clean up environmental pollutants, mitigating soil and water contamination. Moreover, biotechnology enables the production of biofuels, reducing dependence on fossil fuels and curbing greenhouse gas emissions.

In the field of biomedical science, biotechnology has made significant contributions as well. It has facilitated the development of new drugs, vaccines, and diagnostics through techniques such as recombinant DNA technology and gene therapy. Biomedical researchers utilize biotechnology to study the genetic basis of diseases, identify potential drug targets, and develop personalized medicine approaches.

In conclusion, biotechnology is a powerful tool that has revolutionized agriculture and biomedical science. Its applications in agriculture range from genetic modification of crops to improve productivity and nutritional value, to the development of sustainable farming practices. In the field of biomedical science, biotechnology has paved the way for advancements in drug development and personalized medicine. As biotechnology continues to evolve, its potential to address global challenges in agriculture and healthcare remains immense, making it a crucial field for both scientists and the general public to understand.

Genetic Engineering: Manipulating Plant and Animal Genomes

In the realm of biotechnology, genetic engineering holds immense potential for revolutionizing agriculture and food production. By manipulating the genomes of plants and animals, scientists can enhance desired traits, improve crop yields, and develop new varieties that are resistant to pests, diseases, and harsh environmental conditions. This subchapter explores the fascinating field of genetic engineering and its profound implications for the future of farming and food security.

Genetic engineering involves the deliberate modification of an organism's genetic material using various techniques. In the context of agriculture, this technology enables scientists to introduce specific genes into plants and animals, thereby altering their characteristics. For example, by inserting a gene responsible for drought tolerance into a crop, scientists can create drought-resistant varieties that can thrive even in arid regions. Similarly, genetic engineering can be used to enhance the nutritional value of crops, resulting in more nutritious and healthier food options.

One of the significant advantages of genetic engineering is its potential to address global food challenges. With the world's population projected to reach 9 billion by 2050, ensuring food security becomes a crucial priority. Genetic engineering allows scientists to develop crops that can withstand pests and diseases, reducing the need for harmful pesticides and minimizing crop losses. This technology also offers the possibility of developing crops with higher yields, thus increasing food production without expanding agricultural land.

Moreover, genetic engineering is not limited to plants; it also extends to animals. Scientists can modify animal genomes to improve livestock productivity, enhance disease resistance, and even produce pharmaceutical substances in animals. For instance, genetically engineered livestock can be designed to produce therapeutic proteins in their milk, providing a cost-effective and sustainable method of producing life-saving drugs.

However, genetic engineering also raises ethical and environmental concerns. Critics argue that manipulating the natural genetic makeup of organisms may have unforeseen consequences, such as unintended effects on ecosystems or the creation of genetically modified organisms (GMOs) that could pose risks to human health. Addressing these concerns requires strict regulation, thorough risk assessments, and transparent communication between scientists, policymakers, and the public.

In conclusion, genetic engineering represents a powerful tool in the hands of scientists, capable of transforming agriculture and food production. While it offers immense potential for addressing global challenges, it also demands responsible and ethical implementation. As the field of biotechnology advances, understanding the implications of genetic engineering becomes crucial for both the scientific community and the general public.

Crop Improvement through Biotechnology

Biotechnology has revolutionized the field of agriculture and food production, offering innovative solutions to enhance the quality, productivity, and sustainability of crops. This subchapter explores the significant role of biotechnology in crop improvement, highlighting its impact on the global food system.

Biotechnology involves the application of scientific techniques to manipulate the genetic makeup of organisms, including plants, to achieve desired traits. With the advent of biotechnology, scientists have been able to develop genetically modified (GM) crops that possess improved characteristics, such as increased resistance to pests and diseases, enhanced nutritional content, and tolerance to harsh environmental conditions.

One of the key techniques employed in crop improvement through biotechnology is genetic engineering. This process involves the transfer of specific genes from one organism to another, resulting in the expression of desired traits in the recipient plant. For example, scientists have successfully engineered crops to produce their own insecticides, reducing the need for chemical pesticides and minimizing harm to beneficial insects and the environment.

Biotechnology has also played a crucial role in addressing global challenges, such as climate change and food security. By introducing genes that confer drought and salinity tolerance, crops can thrive in arid regions with minimal water availability, ensuring a stable food supply for populations facing water scarcity. Additionally, genetically modified crops with improved nutritional profiles have been developed to combat malnutrition in developing countries.

Moreover, biotechnology has facilitated the development of sustainable farming practices. Through genetic engineering, crops can be engineered to require fewer inputs, such as fertilizers and water, reducing the environmental impact of agricultural activities. This not only minimizes the use of non-renewable resources but also lowers production costs for farmers.

However, it is important to address concerns associated with biotechnology, such as potential environmental risks and ethical considerations. Regulatory frameworks and rigorous safety assessments are in place to ensure the responsible and safe application of biotechnology in agriculture.

In conclusion, biotechnology has revolutionized crop improvement, offering a range of benefits to enhance agricultural productivity, sustainability, and food security. By harnessing the power of genetic engineering, scientists can develop crops with improved traits, contributing to a more resilient and efficient global food system. However, it is crucial to approach biotechnology with caution, ensuring that its application aligns with ethical and environmental considerations.

Livestock Biotechnology: Enhancing Animal Health and Productivity

Livestock biotechnology has revolutionized the field of animal agriculture, leading to significant advancements in animal health and productivity. This subchapter explores how biotechnology has transformed the way we care for and raise livestock, ensuring healthier animals and increased productivity for the benefit of everyone involved in the agricultural and food production industry.

One of the key areas where biotechnology has made a tremendous impact is in the field of animal genetics. Through advanced techniques such as gene editing and genetic engineering, scientists can now manipulate the genetic makeup of animals to enhance desirable traits. This has led to the development of livestock with improved disease resistance, higher milk or meat production, and enhanced nutritional content. By selectively breeding animals with desired traits, farmers can now produce healthier and more productive livestock, ultimately leading to better quality food products for consumers.

Another significant breakthrough in livestock biotechnology is the development of vaccines and diagnostic tools for animal diseases. With the help of biotechnology, scientists can now create vaccines that are more effective, safe, and affordable. These vaccines help prevent diseases such as foot-and-mouth disease, brucellosis, and avian influenza, which have the potential to cause significant losses in the livestock industry. Additionally, biotechnology has enabled the development of rapid and accurate diagnostic tests, allowing for early detection and prompt treatment of diseases, improving animal health and minimizing economic losses.

Biotechnology has also played a crucial role in improving animal nutrition. Through genetic engineering, scientists have developed crops with enhanced nutritional profiles, known as genetically modified organisms (GMOs). These crops can be utilized as animal feed, providing livestock with a more balanced and nutritious diet. In turn, this improves the overall health and productivity of animals.

Furthermore, biotechnology has contributed to the development of growth-promoting hormones and antibiotics used in livestock production. These substances help accelerate growth rates and improve feed efficiency, leading to increased productivity. However, it is essential to ensure responsible and ethical use of these technologies to avoid any negative impact on animal welfare or the environment.

In conclusion, livestock biotechnology has revolutionized animal agriculture, offering immense benefits to both animal health and productivity. By harnessing the power of biotechnology, scientists and farmers can produce healthier animals, develop effective vaccines and diagnostic tools, improve animal nutrition, and enhance the overall efficiency of livestock production. These advancements contribute to a more sustainable and efficient agriculture industry, ensuring a better future for both producers and consumers.

Chapter 3: Biotechnology and Crop Production

Overview of Biotech Crops: GM Crops and their Benefits

Biotechnology has revolutionized the agricultural industry, providing innovative solutions to enhance crop production and address global food security challenges. One of the key advancements in this field is the development of genetically modified (GM) crops, which have gained widespread attention and controversy.

GM crops are plants that have been genetically engineered to possess desirable traits, such as increased resistance to pests, diseases, and environmental stresses, as well as improved nutritional value and shelf life. These crops are created through the insertion of specific genes from other organisms, enabling them to express these desired characteristics.

The benefits of GM crops are numerous and have a significant impact on agricultural practices and food production. Firstly, they offer increased crop yield, allowing farmers to produce more food on limited land. This is particularly crucial in a world where the population is rapidly growing, and arable land is becoming scarce. By improving crop productivity, GM crops contribute to global food security and help feed the expanding population.

Secondly, GM crops can reduce the need for chemical pesticides and herbicides. Many GM crops are engineered to produce their own natural defenses against pests and diseases, reducing the reliance on harmful chemical inputs. This not only benefits the environment by minimizing chemical pollution but also improves the health and safety of farmers and consumers.

Additionally, GM crops can improve the nutritional content of food. For instance, biofortified GM crops, such as Golden Rice, have been developed to combat nutrient deficiencies, providing essential vitamins and minerals in regions where diets may lack these nutrients. This has the potential to alleviate malnutrition and improve public health in vulnerable populations.

Despite these benefits, GM crops have faced criticism and concerns regarding their safety and potential environmental impact. However, extensive research and regulatory processes ensure that GM crops are thoroughly tested and evaluated before commercialization, ensuring their safety for human consumption and the environment.

In conclusion, GM crops are a significant advancement in biotechnology, offering numerous benefits to agriculture and food production. They enhance crop productivity, reduce reliance on chemical inputs, and improve the nutritional content of food. While concerns exist, rigorous safety assessments and regulations ensure the responsible deployment of GM crops. As the world continues to grapple with global food security challenges, GM crops play a crucial role in meeting the growing demand for sustainable and nutritious food.

Herbicide Tolerance: Reducing Weed Pressure in Fields

In modern agriculture, weed management is a crucial aspect of crop production. Weeds compete with crops for essential resources like water, nutrients, and sunlight, leading to significant yield losses. Traditional weed control methods, such as manual weeding or mechanical cultivation, can be time-consuming, labor-intensive, and expensive. However, with the advent of biotechnology, a new and effective tool has emerged to combat weed pressure in fields: herbicide tolerance.

Herbicide tolerance refers to the ability of a crop to withstand the application of specific herbicides, allowing the selective control of weeds while preserving the crop's health and productivity. This trait is achieved through the integration of biotechnology techniques, such as genetic engineering, into crop breeding programs. By introducing genes that encode enzymes capable of detoxifying or degrading herbicides, scientists have been able to develop herbicide-tolerant crops.

The benefits of herbicide tolerance are numerous. Firstly, it provides farmers with a more efficient and cost-effective weed control method. Instead of spending hours manually removing weeds or using heavy machinery for cultivation, farmers can simply apply herbicides to their herbicide-tolerant crops. This not only saves time and labor but also reduces the risk of soil erosion associated with mechanical weed control.

Secondly, herbicide tolerance allows for the use of more environmentally friendly herbicides. With the development of herbicide-tolerant crops, farmers can now use herbicides that specifically target and eliminate weeds while being less harmful to the environment. This targeted approach minimizes the impact on non-target organisms and decreases the overall amount of herbicide required.

Furthermore, herbicide tolerance contributes to sustainable agriculture by reducing the need for multiple herbicide applications. This not only saves costs for farmers but also lowers the potential for herbicide resistance in weed populations. By using herbicide-tolerant crops in rotation with other weed control methods, farmers can effectively manage weed populations and reduce the development of herbicide-resistant weeds.

However, it is important to note that herbicide tolerance should be used as part of an integrated weed management strategy. Crop rotation, cover cropping, and the use of non-chemical weed control methods should also be employed to maintain long-term weed control efficacy and prevent the emergence of resistant weed populations.

In conclusion, herbicide tolerance is a valuable tool in reducing weed pressure in fields. By allowing for efficient and targeted weed control, it improves crop productivity, reduces costs, and minimizes environmental impact. The integration of biotechnology in agriculture through herbicide-tolerant crops showcases the potential of science to revolutionize farming practices and ensure sustainable food production for a growing global population.

Pest Resistance: Enhancing Crop Protection

Introduction:
In our quest to feed a growing global population, agriculture faces numerous challenges, with pests being one of the most significant threats to crop yield. Traditional methods of pest control, such as chemical pesticides, have proven effective, but they come with their own set of concerns. Fortunately, advancements in biotechnology have paved the way for innovative solutions that enhance crop protection by introducing pest resistance into plants themselves.

Understanding Pest Resistance:
Pest resistance refers to the ability of plants to defend themselves against harmful insects, nematodes, or pathogens. By enhancing crop plants with resistance traits, we can reduce the need for chemical pesticides, which can have detrimental effects on humans and the environment. Biotechnology plays a crucial role in developing pest-resistant crops by precisely introducing genetic modifications.

Genetically Modified (GM) Crops:
Genetically modified crops have been engineered to possess specific traits that make them resistant to pests. For example, Bacillus thuringiensis (Bt) genes can be inserted into crop plants, allowing them to produce toxins that are toxic to specific insect pests. This approach has been particularly successful in reducing the damage caused by pests like corn borers and cotton bollworms. By incorporating pest resistance traits into crops, farmers can protect their yields while minimizing the use of harmful pesticides.

Benefits of Pest-Resistant Crops:
The adoption of pest-resistant crops brings numerous benefits. Firstly, it reduces the reliance on chemical pesticide use, which can have adverse effects on human health and the environment. Moreover, pest-resistant crops can lead to higher crop yields, ensuring food security and reducing economic losses for farmers. Additionally, it allows for more sustainable farming practices, preserving biodiversity and minimizing the impact on non-target organisms.

Challenges and Future Directions:
While pest-resistant crops offer significant advantages, it is essential to address the concerns surrounding their use. Some concerns include potential resistance development in pests and the need for careful management strategies to prevent unintended environmental consequences. Additionally, public acceptance and understanding of biotechnology in agriculture play a crucial role in the successful adoption of pest-resistant crops.

Conclusion:
Pest resistance is a critical aspect of crop protection in the face of increasing pest pressure. Biotechnology offers innovative solutions by introducing genetic modifications into crops, enhancing their ability to defend against pests. The adoption of pest-resistant crops brings benefits such as reduced pesticide use, increased crop yields, and more sustainable agricultural practices. However, it is important to address challenges and ensure responsible management to maximize the potential of biotechnology in enhancing crop protection and ensuring food security for everyone.

Drought and Salinity Tolerance: Improving Crop Resilience

In recent years, the world has witnessed the devastating effects of climate change, including frequent droughts and increased soil salinity. These environmental challenges pose significant threats to global food security, as they reduce crop yields and limit agricultural productivity. However, thanks to advancements in biotechnology, scientists have made remarkable progress in developing crops with enhanced drought and salinity tolerance, thereby improving their resilience in the face of these adversities.

Drought is one of the most challenging environmental conditions that crops face. It results in water scarcity, hindering plant growth and development. Traditional breeding techniques have been moderately successful in developing drought-tolerant varieties, but the process is time-consuming and often yields limited results. Biotechnology, on the other hand, offers a faster and more precise approach to enhance crop resilience. Through genetic engineering, scientists can introduce genes that enable plants to conserve water, regulate their water usage, or tolerate prolonged periods of water scarcity. This has led to the development of drought-tolerant crop varieties that can withstand dry spells and maintain acceptable yields even in arid regions.

Similarly, soil salinity poses a significant threat to agriculture, as excessive salt levels negatively impact crop growth and productivity. Biotechnology has played a crucial role in improving crop tolerance to salinity by introducing genes that help plants regulate their salt uptake and maintain cellular balance. Through genetic modification, scientists have successfully developed salt-tolerant crops that can thrive in saline soils, expanding the agricultural potential of previously unusable land and reducing the pressure on fertile areas.

The development and adoption of drought and salinity-tolerant crops have several benefits. Firstly, it ensures food security by reducing the vulnerability of crops to changing climatic conditions. With these resilient varieties, farmers can achieve higher yields even in water-limited or saline environments, ultimately contributing to global food production. Additionally, these biotechnological advancements minimize the need for excessive irrigation, conserving water resources and promoting sustainable agricultural practices. By enhancing crop resilience, biotechnology plays a critical role in mitigating the adverse effects of climate change on food production.

In conclusion, the development of drought and salinity-tolerant crops through biotechnology has revolutionized agriculture and food production. By introducing genes that improve water conservation and salt tolerance, scientists have successfully enhanced the resilience of crops, ensuring food security in the face of climate change. These advancements offer hope for a sustainable future, where crops can thrive even in the harshest environmental conditions. However, it is essential to continue supporting research and development in biotechnology to further improve crop resilience and address the challenges that lie ahead.

Chapter 4: Biotechnology and Livestock Production

Animal Biotechnology: An Overview

Animal biotechnology is a rapidly growing field that has revolutionized the way we understand and interact with animals. It encompasses a wide range of scientific techniques and technologies that are used to improve animal health, welfare, and productivity. From genetic engineering to reproductive technologies, animal biotechnology offers immense potential for advancements in biomedical science and biotechnology.

One of the key areas of focus in animal biotechnology is genetic engineering. This technique involves manipulating an animal's genetic material to introduce desirable traits or remove harmful ones. Genetic engineering has been instrumental in developing animals that are resistant to diseases, such as pigs that are resistant to the deadly viral disease, Porcine Reproductive and Respiratory Syndrome (PRRS). By modifying the animals' genes, scientists have been able to enhance their natural defense mechanisms and improve their overall health.

Reproductive technologies are another crucial aspect of animal biotechnology. These technologies allow scientists to manipulate the reproductive processes of animals, including artificial insemination, embryo transfer, and cloning. For example, in the field of livestock production, artificial insemination has been widely adopted to improve breeding programs and ensure the production of high-quality offspring. Cloning, on the other hand, has opened up new possibilities for preserving endangered species and maintaining genetic diversity.

Animal biotechnology also plays a significant role in the development of pharmaceuticals and biomedical research. Through the use of transgenic animals, scientists can produce human proteins and antibodies that are essential for the development of drugs and vaccines. These genetically modified animals serve as living bioreactors, producing large quantities of valuable substances that can be used for medical purposes.

Furthermore, animal biotechnology has contributed to advancements in the field of regenerative medicine. Stem cell research, for instance, holds great promise in the treatment of diseases and injuries in both animals and humans. By harnessing the power of stem cells, scientists can regenerate damaged tissues and organs, potentially revolutionizing medical treatments and improving the quality of life for many.

In conclusion, animal biotechnology is a dynamic field that encompasses various scientific techniques and technologies aimed at improving animal health, welfare, and productivity. From genetic engineering to reproductive technologies, it offers immense potential for advancements in biomedical science and biotechnology. By harnessing the power of animal biotechnology, we can address critical challenges in agriculture, healthcare, and conservation, paving the way for a more sustainable and prosperous future.

Biotechnological Approaches to Enhancing Animal Health

In recent years, biotechnology has emerged as a powerful tool in the field of agriculture and food production. While much of the focus has been on improving crop yields and developing genetically modified organisms, biotechnological approaches have also been instrumental in enhancing animal health. This subchapter explores the various ways in which biotechnology is revolutionizing the field of veterinary medicine, benefiting both animals and humans alike.

One of the most significant advancements in biotechnology has been the development of vaccines for animals. Vaccines have long been used to prevent and control diseases in humans, and now they are being utilized to protect animals as well. Through genetic engineering, scientists have been able to produce vaccines that are more effective and safer for animals. These vaccines help prevent the spread of infectious diseases among livestock, reducing the need for antibiotics and ultimately improving the safety of the food we consume.

Another biotechnological approach to enhancing animal health is through the development of diagnostic tests. These tests, often based on DNA or protein analysis, allow for the early detection of diseases and the prompt implementation of treatment strategies. By identifying diseases at an early stage, veterinarians can provide appropriate care, minimizing suffering and preventing the spread of contagious illnesses.

Furthermore, genetic engineering has facilitated the production of transgenic animals that are resistant to certain diseases. For example, scientists have successfully developed pigs that are resistant to the devastating African swine fever virus. By introducing specific genes into the animals' DNA, they have effectively created a population that is more resilient to this deadly disease, reducing economic losses and ensuring a stable food supply.

Biotechnology has also played a crucial role in the development of novel therapies for animals. Through genetic modification, scientists have created animals that produce therapeutic proteins in their milk or eggs. These proteins can be harvested and used as treatments for various diseases, such as hemophilia or cystic fibrosis. This approach not only benefits the animals themselves but also provides a sustainable source of medication for human patients.

In conclusion, biotechnological approaches have revolutionized the field of veterinary medicine, enhancing animal health in numerous ways. From the development of vaccines and diagnostic tests to the creation of disease-resistant animals and the production of therapeutic proteins, biotechnology has proven to be a valuable tool in improving the well-being of animals. By utilizing these advancements, we can ensure a healthier and safer food supply while simultaneously improving animal welfare.

Improving Animal Productivity through Biotechnology

Biotechnology has revolutionized the field of agriculture and food production, and one area where its impact has been particularly significant is in improving animal productivity. Through the application of biotechnological techniques, scientists have been able to enhance the genetic makeup of various animal species, resulting in increased productivity, improved health, and more sustainable farming practices.

One of the most widely recognized advancements in animal productivity is the development of genetically modified organisms (GMOs). GMOs have been engineered to possess desirable traits, such as increased resistance to diseases, improved feed efficiency, and enhanced growth rates. These modifications have led to higher meat and milk yields, allowing farmers to produce more food with fewer resources. This has not only helped meet the growing global demand for animal products but has also contributed to more sustainable farming practices by reducing the environmental footprint of livestock production.

In addition to GMOs, biotechnology has also played a crucial role in improving animal health. Researchers have developed vaccines that can be administered to livestock, protecting them from various diseases and reducing the need for antibiotics. This has not only improved the overall health and welfare of animals but has also contributed to a safer and more sustainable food supply. Furthermore, biotechnological advancements have allowed for the development of diagnostic tools that can detect diseases in animals at an early stage, enabling prompt treatment and preventing the spread of contagious illnesses.

Biotechnology has also enabled the production of pharmaceuticals and other valuable products through animal bioreactors. Through genetic engineering, animals can be modified to produce human proteins, enzymes, and antibodies in their milk or blood. These products have significant applications in the field of biomedical science and biotechnology, including the development of new drugs, therapies, and diagnostic tools.

Overall, the application of biotechnology in improving animal productivity has had a transformative impact on agriculture and food production. It has allowed for the production of more food with fewer resources, improved animal health and welfare, and enabled the development of valuable pharmaceuticals. By embracing biotechnological advancements, we can continue to enhance animal productivity, promote sustainable farming practices, and ensure a safe and abundant food supply for future generations.

Biotechnology and Animal Welfare

Animal welfare is a topic of increasing concern in today's society, and the role of biotechnology in addressing these concerns is both significant and promising. Biotechnology, the use of living organisms or their products to improve or develop new technologies, has the potential to revolutionize the way we interact with animals, ensuring their well-being and promoting ethical practices in various sectors, including agriculture and food production.

In the field of biomedicine, biotechnology plays a crucial role in advancing animal welfare. Through genetic engineering, scientists can develop animal models that closely mimic human diseases, enabling the development of new treatments and therapies. By studying these models, researchers can gain a better understanding of diseases and test potential treatments, ultimately leading to improved healthcare outcomes for both humans and animals.

Biotechnology also offers innovative solutions to improve animal health and well-being in agriculture. For instance, genetic engineering can be used to produce animals that are resistant to diseases, reducing the need for antibiotics and other medications. This not only keeps animals healthier but also reduces the risk of antibiotic resistance, benefiting both animal and human health.

Furthermore, biotechnology allows for more sustainable and ethical practices in animal agriculture. By utilizing biotechnological methods, such as in vitro meat production, we can reduce the dependence on traditional livestock farming, which often involves unethical practices like overcrowding and inhumane treatment. In vitro meat, also known as cultured meat, is grown from animal cells in a lab, eliminating the need for animal slaughter and significantly reducing the environmental impact associated with traditional meat production.

In addition to its direct applications, biotechnology also plays a pivotal role in monitoring and ensuring animal welfare standards. For example, biotechnological tools such as DNA analysis can be used to trace the origin of animal products, ensuring that they are sourced from ethical and sustainable farms.

Overall, biotechnology offers immense potential for improving animal welfare across various sectors. By harnessing its power, we can create a more compassionate and sustainable relationship with animals, ensuring their well-being and promoting ethical practices in agriculture and food production. As the field of biotechnology continues to advance, it is crucial for individuals in the biomedical science and biotechnology niches, as well as the general public, to be aware of these advancements and actively support the adoption of biotechnological solutions that prioritize animal welfare.

Chapter 5: Biotechnology and Food Processing

Food Processing and Biotechnology: An Introduction

Food processing and biotechnology play a crucial role in modern agriculture and food production. These two fields are closely interconnected, with biotechnology offering innovative solutions to enhance the efficiency, safety, and sustainability of food processing.

Food processing involves transforming raw agricultural materials into edible products that are safe, nutritious, and appealing to consumers. It encompasses a wide range of activities, including cleaning, sorting, grinding, cooking, packaging, and distribution. The goal is to extend the shelf life of food, minimize waste, and provide convenient and tasty options for consumers.

Biotechnology, on the other hand, involves using living organisms or their components to develop or improve products and processes. In the context of food processing, biotechnology offers tools and techniques that allow scientists to manipulate the genetic makeup of crops, improve crop yields, enhance nutritional content, and develop new varieties with desirable traits.

One of the key applications of biotechnology in food processing is genetic engineering. This technique enables scientists to introduce specific genes into crops, resulting in plants that are resistant to pests, diseases, or environmental stresses. Genetic engineering has been instrumental in developing crops that require fewer pesticides and have enhanced nutritional profiles, such as biofortified crops with increased levels of vitamins or minerals.

Moreover, biotechnology has revolutionized food processing through the use of enzymes and microorganisms. Enzymes are naturally occurring proteins that act as catalysts, speeding up chemical reactions. In food processing, enzymes are used to improve texture, flavor, and nutritional value. For example, enzymes can break down complex carbohydrates into simpler sugars, making them more easily digestible.

Microorganisms, such as bacteria and yeasts, are also employed in food processing. They can ferment ingredients, produce enzymes, or help in the preservation of food. Fermentation is a process that converts sugars into alcohol or organic acids, resulting in the production of various products like bread, cheese, yogurt, and beer.

Overall, food processing and biotechnology are essential for meeting the growing demand for safe, nutritious, and sustainable food. By harnessing the power of biotechnology, scientists and food processors can develop innovative solutions that address challenges such as food security, environmental sustainability, and nutritional deficiencies.

In this book, "From Farm to Lab: The Role of Biotechnology in Agriculture and Food Production," we will explore the fascinating world of food processing and biotechnology. We will delve into the science behind these fields, examine the latest advancements, and discuss their impacts on various aspects of agriculture and food production. Whether you are a student, a researcher, or simply someone interested in the future of our food, this book will provide valuable insights into the role of biotechnology in transforming the way we grow, process, and consume our food.

Microbial Biotechnology: Fermentation and Food Preservation

In the world of agriculture and food production, microbial biotechnology plays a crucial role in ensuring the safety, quality, and longevity of our food supply. One of the most widely used techniques in this field is fermentation, which has been practiced for centuries to enhance the flavor, texture, and nutritional value of various food products.

Fermentation is a natural process that involves the breakdown of complex organic compounds by microorganisms such as bacteria, yeasts, and molds. These microorganisms utilize sugar or other substrates present in the food, converting them into simpler compounds like alcohol, organic acids, or gases. This transformation not only imparts unique flavors and aromas but also increases the shelf life of the food by inhibiting the growth of harmful bacteria.

Cheese, yogurt, bread, beer, and wine are just a few examples of fermented foods that have been enjoyed by humans for centuries. These products undergo controlled fermentation processes, where specific strains of microorganisms are carefully selected and cultivated to achieve desired taste, texture, and nutritional profiles. For instance, the use of specific strains of bacteria in yogurt production not only provides a tangy flavor but also enhances the digestibility of lactose, making it suitable for lactose-intolerant individuals.

Apart from enhancing the sensory attributes of food, fermentation also offers several health benefits. Fermented foods are known to contain probiotics, which are beneficial bacteria that can improve gut health and boost the immune system. Regular consumption of probiotic-rich foods has been linked to improved digestion, reduced risk of certain chronic diseases, and enhanced overall well-being.

In addition to fermentation, microbial biotechnology also plays a vital role in food preservation. Preservation techniques aim to extend the shelf life of food products by inhibiting the growth of spoilage-causing microorganisms and preventing foodborne illnesses. One such technique is the use of lactic acid bacteria to produce lactic acid, which creates an acidic environment that inhibits the growth of harmful bacteria.

Furthermore, the use of microbial biotechnology in food preservation has led to the development of novel techniques such as biopreservation and the use of antimicrobial peptides. Biopreservation involves the use of beneficial microorganisms or their metabolic products to prevent the growth of pathogens and spoilage organisms. Antimicrobial peptides, on the other hand, are naturally occurring compounds produced by microorganisms that can effectively kill or inhibit the growth of harmful bacteria.

Microbial biotechnology, through fermentation and food preservation techniques, offers a wide range of benefits to both the industry and consumers. It not only enhances the sensory attributes and nutritional value of food but also ensures its safety and extends its shelf life. By harnessing the power of microorganisms, we can continue to enjoy a diverse and sustainable food supply while promoting the health and well-being of individuals worldwide.

Genetic Modification in Food Processing: Enhancing Nutritional Value

In the ever-evolving field of biotechnology, genetic modification has emerged as a powerful tool to enhance the nutritional value of food through the manipulation of genetic material. This subchapter explores the role of genetic modification in food processing and its potential to address nutritional deficiencies and improve human health.

Genetic modification involves the intentional alteration of an organism's genetic material to impart specific traits or characteristics. In the context of food processing, it allows scientists to introduce or enhance certain desirable traits in crops, such as increased nutrient content, improved taste, and extended shelf life.

One of the most significant applications of genetic modification in food processing is the enhancement of nutritional value. By introducing genes that encode essential nutrients, scientists can fortify crops with vitamins, minerals, and other beneficial compounds. For example, rice has been genetically modified to produce beta-carotene, a precursor of vitamin A, addressing vitamin A deficiency in regions where rice is a staple food.

Genetic modification also enables the reduction of anti-nutritional factors present in some crops. Anti-nutrients are compounds that interfere with the absorption of essential nutrients, limiting their bioavailability. Through genetic modification, these compounds can be minimized, making the nutrients more accessible and beneficial for human consumption.

Furthermore, genetic modification can improve the quality and safety of processed foods. For instance, genetically modified crops can be engineered to resist pests and diseases, reducing the need for chemical pesticides. This not only benefits human health but also minimizes environmental impacts associated with conventional agriculture.

It is important to note that the advancements in genetic modification are subject to rigorous safety assessments and regulations. Extensive research is conducted to ensure that genetically modified foods are safe for human consumption, with regulatory bodies closely monitoring their development and commercialization.

While genetic modification in food processing holds tremendous potential, it is essential to address concerns and engage in open dialogue. Transparency and clear labeling are crucial to provide consumers with information about genetically modified ingredients, allowing them to make informed choices.

In conclusion, genetic modification in food processing represents a powerful tool to enhance nutritional value, improve food quality, and address nutritional deficiencies. Through the intentional alteration of genetic material, scientists can fortify crops with essential nutrients, reduce anti-nutritional factors, and enhance food safety. However, it is crucial to approach genetic modification with caution, ensuring rigorous safety assessments and transparent communication with consumers. By harnessing the potential of genetic modification, we can pave the way for a more sustainable and nutritious future in agriculture and food production.

(Note: The content above provides a brief summary of the subchapter "Genetic Modification in Food Processing: Enhancing Nutritional Value" from the book "From Farm to Lab: The Role of Biotechnology in Agriculture and Food Production". It is designed to address a broad audience, including those interested in Biomedical Science and Biotechnology.)

Chapter 6: Biotechnology and Food Safety

Ensuring Food Safety: An Introduction to Biotechnology

Biotechnology has revolutionized the agricultural and food production industries, playing a crucial role in ensuring food safety. This subchapter provides an introduction to the use of biotechnology in these sectors and highlights its significance in safeguarding the health and well-being of consumers.

Biotechnology encompasses a range of scientific techniques that utilize living organisms or their components to develop new products or improve existing ones. In the context of agriculture and food production, biotechnology offers innovative solutions to enhance crop yields, improve nutritional content, and most importantly, ensure food safety.

One of the key applications of biotechnology in food safety is the development of genetically modified organisms (GMOs). Through genetic engineering, scientists can introduce specific traits into plants or animals, making them more resistant to pests, diseases, or environmental conditions. This not only increases crop productivity but also reduces the reliance on chemical pesticides and fertilizers, minimizing their potential negative impacts on human health and the environment.

Another significant aspect of biotechnology in food safety is the use of molecular diagnostics. These techniques enable the rapid and accurate detection of foodborne pathogens, allergens, and other contaminants. By identifying and monitoring the presence of harmful substances in food products, biotechnology helps prevent outbreaks of foodborne illnesses and ensures the timely withdrawal of contaminated products from the market.

Furthermore, biotechnology plays a critical role in food preservation and processing. Techniques such as genetic modification, irradiation, and enzymatic treatments can extend the shelf life of perishable food items while maintaining their nutritional value and sensory properties. This not only reduces food waste but also enhances food safety by inhibiting the growth of spoilage microorganisms and reducing the risk of foodborne infections.

It is essential for individuals in the fields of biomedical science and biotechnology to stay informed about the latest advancements and ethical considerations surrounding biotechnology in the context of food safety. Understanding the potential benefits and risks associated with genetically modified foods, molecular diagnostics, and food processing techniques empowers scientists and policymakers to make informed decisions and ensure the safety and quality of the food we consume.

In conclusion, biotechnology plays a vital role in ensuring food safety. From genetically modified crops to molecular diagnostics and food preservation techniques, biotechnology offers innovative solutions to enhance productivity, detect contaminants, and extend shelf life. By staying informed about the advancements in this field, individuals in the niches of biomedical science and biotechnology can contribute to the development and implementation of safe and sustainable agricultural and food production practices.

Biotechnology and Foodborne Pathogens: Detection and Control

The safety and quality of our food are of paramount importance, as they directly impact our health and well-being. In recent years, the emergence and spread of foodborne pathogens have posed significant challenges to the agricultural and food production sectors. Biotechnology, with its innovative approaches, has emerged as a key player in the detection and control of these pathogens, ensuring the safety and integrity of our food supply chain.

Detecting foodborne pathogens is a crucial step in preventing foodborne illnesses. Traditional methods of detection often require time-consuming and labor-intensive processes, resulting in delayed response times and increased risks. Biotechnology has revolutionized pathogen detection by introducing rapid and highly sensitive techniques. These methods employ advanced molecular tools, such as polymerase chain reaction (PCR) and DNA microarrays, which can quickly identify the presence of specific pathogens in food samples. By significantly reducing the detection time, biotechnology enables prompt actions to prevent contaminated products from reaching consumers.

Once foodborne pathogens are detected, effective control measures must be implemented to ensure consumer safety. Biotechnology offers a range of innovative strategies for pathogen control. One such approach is the use of bacteriophages, which are viruses that specifically target and destroy harmful bacteria. These natural predators of bacteria can be applied directly to food products or used in sanitizing agents to eliminate pathogens without affecting the taste, color, or texture of the food.

Another promising biotechnological solution is the development of genetically modified organisms (GMOs) with enhanced resistance to foodborne pathogens. Through genetic engineering, scientists can introduce specific genes into crops, making them less susceptible to contamination. For example, researchers have successfully engineered tomatoes that produce antimicrobial peptides, which inhibit the growth of common foodborne pathogens like Salmonella and E. coli. These GMOs have the potential to significantly reduce the risk of foodborne illnesses by minimizing the presence of pathogens in the agricultural environment.

The integration of biotechnology in the detection and control of foodborne pathogens holds great promise for ensuring food safety and reducing the incidence of foodborne illnesses. However, it is essential to strike a balance between technological advancements and ethical considerations, ensuring that these innovative solutions are safe, socially acceptable, and environmentally sustainable. With continued research and development in the field of biotechnology, we can look forward to a future where our food supply is safer, healthier, and more resilient than ever before.

Controversies and Concerns: GMO Labeling and Consumer Awareness

In recent years, the topic of genetically modified organisms (GMOs) has sparked heated debates and raised concerns among consumers worldwide. As the use of biotechnology in agriculture and food production continues to grow, so does the need for transparency and consumer awareness regarding GMOs. This subchapter aims to shed light on the controversies surrounding GMO labeling and the importance of consumer education in the fields of biomedical science and biotechnology.

One of the main controversies surrounding GMOs is the lack of mandatory labeling in many countries. Advocates argue that consumers have the right to know whether the products they purchase contain genetically modified ingredients. They believe that GMO labeling allows individuals to make informed choices about the food they consume and promotes transparency in the food industry. On the other hand, opponents argue that mandatory labeling could create unnecessary panic and misinformation, as GMOs have been extensively tested and found to be safe for consumption.

Consumer awareness plays a crucial role in navigating this controversial landscape. With the growing influence of social media and the internet, it is vital for individuals to be well-informed about GMOs and the scientific evidence surrounding their safety. Biomedical scientists and biotechnologists have a unique opportunity to educate the public about the benefits and risks associated with GMOs, ensuring that consumers have accurate information to base their decisions on.

However, bridging the gap between scientific research and public understanding is not always easy. The complex nature of biotechnology and genetic engineering can be challenging to communicate effectively to a broader audience. It is crucial for experts in the field to engage in science communication and outreach activities, such as public lectures, workshops, and online resources, to promote understanding and dispel misconceptions about GMOs.

Furthermore, collaboration between scientists, policymakers, and consumer advocacy groups is essential in addressing the concerns surrounding GMOs. By fostering open dialogue and sharing information, stakeholders can work together to establish regulations and guidelines that balance the need for transparency with the promotion of scientific literacy.

In conclusion, GMO labeling and consumer awareness are hot topics in the fields of biomedical science and biotechnology. While controversies exist, it is vital to recognize the importance of transparent information and consumer choice. Scientists and experts play a crucial role in educating the public, dispelling myths, and fostering a constructive dialogue to ensure a well-informed society capable of making informed decisions about the food they consume.

Chapter 7: Biotechnology and Sustainable Agriculture

Sustainable Agriculture: An Overview

In today's world, where environmental concerns are at the forefront of global discussions, the concept of sustainable agriculture has gained significant attention. This subchapter aims to provide an overview of sustainable agriculture and its role in addressing the challenges faced by the agricultural industry. Whether you are a curious individual, a student of biomedical science, or someone interested in biotechnology, this information will offer valuable insights into the intersection of sustainable agriculture and biotechnology.

Sustainable agriculture refers to the practice of cultivating food, fiber, and other agricultural products while preserving the environment, safeguarding public health, and ensuring economic profitability for farmers. It emphasizes the use of environmentally friendly practices that maintain soil fertility, conserve water resources, and minimize the use of synthetic chemicals. By adopting sustainable agricultural methods, we can mitigate the negative impacts of conventional farming practices on the environment, such as soil erosion, water pollution, and biodiversity loss.

Biotechnology plays a crucial role in sustainable agriculture by offering innovative solutions to some of the challenges faced by traditional farming systems. Through the application of biotechnology tools, scientists can develop genetically modified crops that are resistant to pests, diseases, and adverse environmental conditions. These genetically modified organisms (GMOs) have the potential to increase crop yields, reduce the reliance on chemical pesticides, and enhance nutritional content.

Moreover, biotechnology enables the development of precision agriculture techniques that optimize resource utilization and minimize waste. By utilizing sensors, drones, and data analytics, farmers can monitor crop health, soil fertility, and water usage in real-time, allowing for targeted interventions and optimized resource allocation. This integration of biotechnology into agriculture not only improves productivity but also reduces the environmental footprint of farming practices.

In addition to biotechnology, sustainable agriculture encompasses other practices such as organic farming, agroforestry, and crop rotation. These practices promote biodiversity, enhance soil fertility, and reduce greenhouse gas emissions. By adopting a holistic approach to agriculture, we can create a more resilient and sustainable food production system that can meet the needs of a growing global population without compromising the health of our planet.

In conclusion, sustainable agriculture is an essential aspect of addressing the environmental and food security challenges of the 21st century. By integrating biotechnology with sustainable farming practices, we can achieve higher yields, reduce the use of chemical inputs, and promote environmental stewardship. This subchapter provides a glimpse into the world of sustainable agriculture and its intersection with biotechnology, offering valuable insights to individuals interested in biomedical science, biotechnology, or anyone passionate about creating a more sustainable future for agriculture and food production.

Biotechnology and Environmental Sustainability

In recent years, biotechnology has emerged as a powerful tool in addressing the global challenges of environmental sustainability. With its ability to harness the potential of living organisms, biotechnology offers innovative solutions to some of the most pressing environmental issues we face today. This subchapter explores the intersection of biotechnology and environmental sustainability, highlighting the role it plays in advancing the fields of agriculture and food production.

One of the key contributions of biotechnology to environmental sustainability lies in its ability to enhance crop productivity while reducing the environmental impact of agriculture. Through genetic engineering, scientists can develop crops that are more resistant to pests, diseases, and harsh environmental conditions. These genetically modified organisms (GMOs) not only ensure higher yields, but also reduce the need for harmful pesticides and herbicides, thus minimizing the negative impact on the environment and human health.

Furthermore, biotechnology offers a promising solution to the global challenge of food scarcity. By developing crops with improved nutritional content and enhanced tolerance to adverse conditions, biotechnologists are working towards ensuring food security for the growing global population. This not only addresses the immediate needs of hunger-stricken regions but also contributes to the long-term sustainability of agricultural practices.

Biotechnology also plays a vital role in environmental conservation and restoration. Through applications such as bioremediation, scientists are using living organisms to clean up and detoxify polluted environments. Microorganisms can be engineered to break down harmful pollutants, such as oil spills or heavy metals, into less harmful substances, thus aiding in the restoration of ecosystems and protecting biodiversity.

Moreover, biotechnology is instrumental in the development of sustainable biofuels. By harnessing the power of microorganisms and plants, scientists can produce biofuels that are renewable, carbon-neutral, and environmentally friendly. These biofuels have the potential to replace fossil fuels, reducing greenhouse gas emissions and mitigating climate change.

In conclusion, biotechnology plays a crucial role in advancing environmental sustainability. By harnessing the potential of living organisms, biotechnologists are developing innovative solutions to address the challenges of agriculture, food production, environmental conservation, and climate change. The applications of biotechnology in these areas not only ensure a more sustainable future but also contribute to the well-being of our planet and all its inhabitants.

Biotechnology and Resource Conservation

In today's world, where the demand for food and resources continues to rise, it has become crucial to find sustainable solutions to ensure the well-being of our planet and its inhabitants. One field that holds immense promise in this regard is biotechnology. Biotechnology, with its ability to harness the power of living organisms and their cellular components, is revolutionizing agriculture and food production, offering innovative ways to conserve resources and protect the environment.

Biotechnology offers numerous tools and techniques that help optimize the use of resources, such as water, energy, and land. Through the application of genetic engineering, scientists can develop crops that require less water or are more resistant to pests and diseases, reducing the need for excessive water usage and chemical pesticides. This not only conserves precious resources but also minimizes the negative environmental impact associated with conventional farming practices.

One of the most significant contributions of biotechnology to resource conservation is the development of genetically modified organisms (GMOs). GMOs are organisms whose genetic material has been altered through biotechnology to exhibit specific traits. In agriculture, GMOs have been engineered to possess desirable characteristics, such as drought resistance or enhanced nutrient content, making them more efficient and sustainable. By using GMOs, farmers can produce higher yields with fewer resources and less environmental impact.

Biotechnology also plays a crucial role in waste management and recycling. Through the use of microorganisms, scientists can develop bioremediation techniques that help clean up polluted environments by breaking down harmful substances into harmless byproducts. Additionally, biotechnology enables the production of biofuels from renewable resources, reducing our reliance on fossil fuels and mitigating climate change.

The field of biotechnology offers immense potential for resource conservation in the biomedical science and biotechnology niches as well. Researchers are developing innovative methods to produce pharmaceuticals, vaccines, and other medical products using biotechnological tools. By optimizing production processes and reducing waste, biotechnology helps conserve resources while ensuring a steady supply of life-saving medications.

In conclusion, biotechnology holds the key to sustainable resource conservation in agriculture, food production, and the biomedical sciences. Its ability to optimize resource utilization, develop genetically modified organisms, and address waste management challenges is invaluable. By embracing biotechnology, we can protect our environment, secure our food supply, and advance medical research, all while ensuring a brighter future for generations to come.

Biotechnology and Organic Farming

In recent years, the world has witnessed a growing interest in sustainable and environmentally friendly agricultural practices. As concerns over the impact of conventional farming methods on the environment and human health have increased, the focus has shifted towards alternative approaches such as organic farming. At the same time, advancements in biotechnology have opened up new possibilities for improving agricultural productivity and sustainability. In this subchapter, we explore the intersection of biotechnology and organic farming and how these two fields can work together to address the challenges facing our global food system.

Organic farming is a holistic approach to agriculture that emphasizes the use of natural inputs and methods to enhance soil fertility, control pests and diseases, and promote overall ecosystem health. It prohibits the use of synthetic pesticides, genetically modified organisms (GMOs), and chemical fertilizers. The organic movement has gained significant momentum in recent years due to its perceived benefits for human health, environmental conservation, and animal welfare. However, organic farming also faces challenges, such as lower yields and increased susceptibility to certain pests and diseases.

Biotechnology, on the other hand, harnesses the power of living organisms and their components to develop innovative solutions for various industries, including agriculture. Biotechnology tools, such as genetic engineering, can enhance crop traits by introducing genes that confer resistance to pests, diseases, or environmental stress. These genetically modified crops, often referred to as GMOs, have been a subject of intense debate. However, the potential benefits they offer, such as increased yields, reduced pesticide use, and improved nutritional content, cannot be ignored.

The integration of biotechnology and organic farming might seem contradictory at first. However, many scientists and farmers believe that combining the two approaches could result in a more sustainable and resilient agricultural system. For instance, biotechnology can help organic farmers address some of the limitations they face, such as pest and disease control. By developing GMOs that are resistant to specific pests or diseases, organic farmers can reduce their reliance on chemical pesticides and still maintain their organic certification.

Furthermore, biotechnology can contribute to organic farming by improving crop nutrition and soil health. Scientists are exploring the use of genetically modified microorganisms to enhance nutrient availability and promote the decomposition of organic matter in the soil. These innovations have the potential to address the nutrient deficiencies often observed in organic farming systems and improve overall crop productivity.

It is important to note that the integration of biotechnology and organic farming should be approached with caution and in accordance with strict regulations and safety protocols. Transparency and clear labeling are also crucial to allow consumers to make informed choices about the food they consume.

In conclusion, the combination of biotechnology and organic farming holds great promise for addressing the challenges facing our agricultural system. By leveraging the benefits of both fields, we can develop sustainable and environmentally friendly practices that ensure food security and promote the well-being of both humans and the planet.

Chapter 8: Future Trends and Challenges in Biotechnology

Emerging Technologies in Biotechnology

In recent years, the field of biotechnology has witnessed remarkable advancements, with emerging technologies revolutionizing various aspects of biomedical science and biotechnology. These cutting-edge technologies hold immense potential to reshape the way we approach agriculture and food production. In this subchapter, we will explore some of the most promising emerging technologies in biotechnology and their significance in the realms of biomedical science and biotechnology.

One such technology that has garnered significant attention is gene editing. Gene editing tools like CRISPR-Cas9 have revolutionized the ability to modify genes with unprecedented precision. This breakthrough technology allows scientists to edit the DNA of organisms, including plants and animals, opening up possibilities for enhanced crop yields, disease-resistant livestock, and improved nutritional content in food. The potential applications of gene editing are vast and hold promise for addressing global challenges related to food security and sustainable agriculture.

Another emerging technology that holds tremendous potential is bioinformatics. With the exponential growth of biological data, bioinformatics plays a crucial role in managing, analyzing, and interpreting this vast amount of information. It enables scientists to make sense of complex biological systems, study genetic variations, and identify potential targets for drug development. Bioinformatics also plays a pivotal role in personalized medicine, allowing healthcare professionals to tailor treatments based on an individual's genetic makeup.

The field of synthetic biology is another area that has gained traction in recent years. Synthetic biology combines biology, engineering, and computer science to design and construct new biological parts, devices, and systems. By engineering organisms to perform specific functions, synthetic biology offers exciting possibilities in areas such as drug production, biofuel development, and environmental remediation. This interdisciplinary field has the potential to revolutionize various industries and contribute to a more sustainable future.

Nanotechnology, with its ability to manipulate matter at the nanoscale, has also emerged as a transformative technology in biotechnology. Nanoparticles and nanosensors are being used for targeted drug delivery, detection of diseases at an early stage, and the development of novel diagnostic tools. The integration of nanotechnology with biotechnology has the potential to revolutionize healthcare and improve patient outcomes.

These are just a few examples of the emerging technologies that are poised to shape the future of biotechnology. As these technologies continue to evolve, it is essential for researchers, policymakers, and the general public to stay informed about their potential benefits and ethical considerations. By embracing these advancements, we can harness the power of biotechnology to address pressing challenges, improve human health, and ensure sustainable agricultural practices.

Ethical Considerations in Biotechnology

In the rapidly advancing field of biotechnology, there are various ethical considerations that need to be taken into account. Biotechnology has the potential to revolutionize agriculture and food production, but it also poses significant ethical dilemmas that must be addressed. This subchapter explores some of the key ethical considerations in biotechnology and highlights the importance of responsible decision-making.

One of the primary ethical considerations in biotechnology is the potential for unintended consequences. Genetic modification, for example, can have unforeseen effects on ecosystems and biodiversity. It is essential to carefully evaluate the potential risks and benefits associated with any biotechnological application to ensure that the overall impact is positive and sustainable.

Additionally, the issue of informed consent and transparency is crucial in biotechnology. When conducting research involving human subjects or genetically modified organisms, it is imperative to obtain informed consent from all parties involved. This ensures that individuals fully understand the potential risks and benefits and have the right to make informed decisions regarding their participation.

Another ethical concern in biotechnology is the equitable distribution of its benefits. Biotechnological advancements have the potential to significantly improve crop yields, enhance nutritional content, and reduce the use of pesticides. However, it is essential to ensure that these benefits reach all segments of society, especially the marginalized and vulnerable populations. Access to biotechnological innovations should not be limited by economic or social factors, but rather should be made available to all individuals, regardless of their socio-economic status.

Furthermore, the issue of biosecurity and biosafety cannot be overlooked. Biotechnology has the potential to create dangerous pathogens or other organisms that could be used for malicious purposes. It is crucial to establish rigorous safety protocols and regulations to prevent the misuse of biotechnological advancements.

Lastly, the ethics of intellectual property rights and patenting in biotechnology should be carefully considered. While patents incentivize innovation and investment in research, they can also hinder the availability and affordability of life-saving technologies. Striking a balance between protecting intellectual property rights and ensuring access to essential biotechnological advancements is of paramount importance.

In conclusion, ethical considerations are an integral part of the biotechnology field. Responsible decision-making, transparency, equitable distribution of benefits, biosecurity, and intellectual property rights all play a significant role in shaping the future of biotechnology. As the field continues to advance, it is crucial for scientists, policymakers, and the public to engage in thoughtful discussions and debates to ensure that biotechnological advancements are used ethically and responsibly to benefit society as a whole.

Regulatory Frameworks: Balancing Innovation and Safety

In the fast-paced world of biotechnology, where advancements are being made at an unprecedented rate, it is crucial to establish regulatory frameworks that strike a delicate balance between fostering innovation and ensuring safety. This subchapter aims to explore the importance of regulatory frameworks in the field of biotechnology, specifically in agriculture and food production, and how they impact both the general audience and the niches of biomedical science and biotechnology.

Biotechnology has revolutionized the way we approach agriculture and food production, offering innovative solutions to enhance crop yields, improve nutritional content, and develop disease-resistant plants. However, along with these exciting advancements comes the need for careful oversight and regulation to address potential risks and maintain public trust.

For the general audience, regulatory frameworks play a vital role in ensuring that the products they consume are safe, reliable, and sustainable. These frameworks set standards for product quality, labeling, and risk assessment, providing consumers with the necessary information to make informed choices about the food they eat. By establishing clear guidelines, regulations help build confidence in biotechnological innovations and their potential benefits.

In the niches of biomedical science and biotechnology, regulatory frameworks are equally crucial. Researchers and scientists working in these fields heavily rely on regulatory agencies to guide their work and ensure ethical practices. Regulations surrounding the use of genetically modified organisms (GMOs) or gene-editing techniques, for instance, help maintain the integrity of research and prevent any potential harm to human health or the environment.

Furthermore, regulatory frameworks also serve as a bridge between industry, academia, and the public. They facilitate communication and collaboration between stakeholders, allowing for the exchange of knowledge, expertise, and concerns. By involving various parties in the regulatory process, these frameworks ensure that innovative biotechnological solutions are developed in a responsible and inclusive manner.

While the regulatory landscape can be complex, it is essential for all stakeholders to understand and engage with these frameworks. By doing so, we can collectively navigate the challenges and opportunities of biotechnology, harnessing its potential while safeguarding public health and environmental sustainability.

In conclusion, regulatory frameworks are indispensable in the realm of biotechnology, playing a crucial role in balancing innovation and safety. They provide the general audience with confidence in the products they consume, while guiding researchers and scientists in their work. By fostering collaboration and transparency, regulatory frameworks pave the way for responsible and sustainable biotechnological advancements that benefit society as a whole.

Overcoming Challenges: Bridging the Gap between Science and Society

In today's fast-paced world, advancements in science and technology are transforming every aspect of our lives. Biotechnology, particularly in the field of agriculture and food production, has revolutionized the way we grow crops, develop medicines, and address global challenges such as hunger and disease. However, despite the tremendous potential of biotechnology, there exists a persistent gap between scientific advancements and their understanding and acceptance by society at large.

This subchapter aims to explore the challenges that arise when bridging the gap between science and society, with a specific focus on the field of biotechnology. Whether you are an individual curious about the latest scientific breakthroughs or a professional in the biomedical science and biotechnology niche, understanding this gap is crucial for progress and informed decision-making.

One of the primary challenges in bridging this gap is the lack of knowledge and understanding about biotechnology among the general public. Misconceptions, fear, and skepticism often arise due to the complexity of the science involved, leading to a hesitancy to embrace new technologies. Therefore, it becomes essential to communicate scientific advancements in a clear, accessible, and relatable manner to engage and educate a wider audience.

Furthermore, ethical concerns surrounding biotechnology can hinder its acceptance. Issues such as genetically modified organisms (GMOs), gene editing, and stem cell research raise questions about the potential risks and benefits. Engaging in open, transparent, and inclusive discussions is necessary to address these concerns and foster a sense of trust between the scientific community and society.

In addition to knowledge and ethical concerns, the economic implications of biotechnology can also pose challenges. While biotechnology has the potential to alleviate global challenges, it may also disrupt traditional agricultural and food production systems. Balancing the need for innovation and progress with the preservation of livelihoods and local economies is a delicate task that requires collaboration between different stakeholders.

To overcome these challenges, it is crucial for scientists, policymakers, educators, and communicators to work together. Public engagement initiatives, science communication programs, and interdisciplinary collaborations can play a significant role in bridging the gap between science and society. By fostering dialogue, understanding, and trust, we can ensure that the benefits of biotechnology are realized and shared by all.

In conclusion, bridging the gap between science and society in the field of biotechnology is a complex and ongoing endeavor. By addressing challenges related to knowledge gaps, ethics, and economic implications, we can create a more inclusive and informed society. Through collaboration and open dialogue, we can overcome these challenges and unlock the full potential of biotechnology to address global challenges and improve the quality of life for everyone.

Chapter 9: Conclusion

Recapitulation of Key Points

In this subchapter, we will summarize the important concepts and key points discussed throughout the book "From Farm to Lab: The Role of Biotechnology in Agriculture and Food Production." This recapitulation aims to provide a comprehensive overview for the general audience, as well as individuals interested in the fields of biomedical science and biotechnology.

Firstly, we explored the fundamental definitions and principles of biotechnology, highlighting its significant role in transforming agriculture and food production. Biotechnology encompasses a wide range of techniques and technologies that utilize living organisms or their components to develop innovative solutions for various challenges in these industries.

We then delved into the benefits of biotechnology in agriculture, emphasizing its potential to increase crop yields, enhance nutritional content, and improve resistance to pests, diseases, and environmental stressors. Through genetic modification and engineering, scientists can create crops with desirable traits, such as drought tolerance or increased vitamin content, ultimately contributing to global food security.

Moreover, we discussed the safety and regulatory aspects of biotechnology. Rigorous testing, risk assessment, and regulatory frameworks ensure that biotech products are safe for human consumption and the environment. The book emphasized the importance of scientific consensus and evidence-based decision-making in this field.

Another key point covered was the impact of biotechnology on sustainable farming practices. By reducing the need for chemical inputs, biotechnology promotes environmentally friendly farming methods. Additionally, we explored the potential of biotechnology in addressing climate change challenges, such as developing crops with increased carbon sequestration capabilities.

Furthermore, we highlighted the role of biotechnology in improving health and medicine. Biomedical science relies on biotechnology to develop novel drugs, diagnostic tools, and therapies. Genetic engineering techniques have revolutionized medical research, enabling the production of life-saving pharmaceuticals and personalized medicine approaches.

Lastly, we emphasized the importance of public understanding and engagement with biotechnology. Education and awareness play a crucial role in fostering informed discussions and decision-making regarding the use of biotechnology in agriculture and food production. By actively participating in the dialogue, individuals can contribute to shaping policies that balance innovation, safety, and sustainability.

In conclusion, "From Farm to Lab: The Role of Biotechnology in Agriculture and Food Production" has provided an overview of the vast potential and benefits of biotechnology in these industries. By harnessing the power of living organisms, scientists can create sustainable farming practices, enhance food security, and improve human health. This book encourages individuals from all backgrounds to engage in the discussion surrounding biotechnology and its applications, fostering a better understanding of its importance and potential.

The Future of Biotechnology in Agriculture and Food Production

In recent years, biotechnology has emerged as a game-changer in the field of agriculture and food production. With advancements in genetic engineering, scientists have been able to enhance crop yields, develop disease-resistant plants, and improve the nutritional content of our food. As we look ahead, the future of biotechnology in agriculture holds tremendous promise for addressing some of the most pressing challenges facing our planet.

One of the key areas where biotechnology is set to revolutionize agriculture is in the development of genetically modified organisms (GMOs). GMOs are created by inserting specific genes into the DNA of plants, giving them desirable traits such as resistance to pests or tolerance to harsh environmental conditions. This technology has the potential to significantly increase agricultural productivity, ensuring food security for a growing global population.

Moreover, biotechnology is helping to reduce the environmental impact of agriculture. By developing crops that require fewer pesticides or fertilizers, we can minimize the negative effects of chemical runoff on ecosystems. Additionally, biotechnological advancements have paved the way for the production of biofuels, which offer a renewable and sustainable alternative to fossil fuels, reducing greenhouse gas emissions and combating climate change.

Biotechnology also plays a crucial role in improving the nutritional value of our food. Scientists are working on developing biofortified crops that are enriched with essential vitamins and minerals, addressing malnutrition in regions where access to a diverse diet is limited. This has the potential to significantly improve public health and reduce the burden of diseases associated with nutrient deficiencies.

Furthermore, biotechnology is revolutionizing the way we produce and consume food. The development of lab-grown meat, for instance, has the potential to transform the livestock industry by reducing the need for traditional animal farming. This not only addresses ethical concerns surrounding animal welfare but also reduces the environmental impact associated with livestock production, such as deforestation and greenhouse gas emissions.

In conclusion, the future of biotechnology in agriculture and food production is filled with immense possibilities. From enhancing crop yields and developing disease-resistant plants to improving the nutritional content of our food and revolutionizing the way we produce and consume it, biotechnology holds the key to a sustainable and secure food future. As we move forward, it is crucial for scientists, policymakers, and the public to collaborate and embrace the potential of biotechnology to address the challenges that lie ahead.

Final Thoughts: Harnessing the Potential of Biotechnology for a Sustainable Future

In the rapidly advancing field of biotechnology, the potential for innovation and progress is immense. From improving crop yields and disease resistance in agriculture to revolutionizing medical treatments and drug development, biotechnology has the power to shape a sustainable future for all. This final chapter aims to highlight the vast possibilities and challenges that lie ahead, encouraging readers from all walks of life, especially those interested in biomedical science and biotechnology, to actively participate in harnessing its potential.

Biotechnology has already made significant contributions to agriculture and food production. Through genetic engineering, scientists have developed crops that are more resistant to pests, diseases, and environmental stressors. This has not only increased crop yields but also reduced the need for harmful pesticides and herbicides, promoting more sustainable farming practices. Additionally, biotechnology has facilitated the production of high-quality and nutritionally enhanced food products, addressing global malnutrition challenges.

In the field of medicine, biotechnology has revolutionized the way we approach disease prevention, diagnosis, and treatment. Advances in genetic engineering and gene editing technologies have paved the way for personalized medicine, tailoring treatments to an individual's genetic makeup. This has the potential to enhance the efficacy of treatments, reduce side effects, and ultimately improve patient outcomes. Biotechnology has also played a crucial role in the development of vaccines, antibiotics, and other life-saving drugs, contributing to the eradication and control of diseases worldwide.

However, as we explore the immense potential of biotechnology, it is crucial to address the ethical, social, and environmental implications associated with its applications. The responsible and sustainable use of biotechnology requires careful regulation, transparency, and public engagement. It is essential to ensure equitable access to biotechnological advancements and consider the potential impact on biodiversity, ecosystems, and traditional farming practices.

To fully harness the potential of biotechnology, it is crucial for individuals from all backgrounds to engage with the field. Whether you are a scientist, a student, a farmer, or a consumer, your participation is vital. Stay informed about the latest developments, ask questions, and participate in discussions surrounding the ethical, social, and environmental dimensions of biotechnology. By doing so, you can contribute to shaping policies, encouraging responsible innovation, and ensuring that biotechnology is used for the collective benefit of humanity and the planet.

In conclusion, biotechnology holds immense promise for a sustainable future in agriculture and healthcare. By embracing its potential while addressing the associated challenges, we can create a world where food security is enhanced, diseases are prevented and treated more effectively, and the environment is protected. The future of biotechnology lies in the hands of all individuals, and it is up to us to harness its potential responsibly for the benefit of present and future generations.